Les Techniques
Danielle Gagné

Zapping
Self-Love

Coloring Book 1

**Self-Care, Self-Love,
and Shiatsu Exercises**

Design and Layout: MJ Schwader
Editor: MJ Schwader

ISBN-13: 978-1973809432
ISBN-10: 1973809435

Dedication

To my beloved mother Mireille Gagné, to whom I offer all the honor of this book.

Acknowledgments

Stylist Linda Morisset: Designer Les Productions Linda Morisset.

Consultant Nikkea B Devida: Expert on accelerated results.

Writing Coach MJ Schwader: Editor, Design and Layout of Cover and Interior.

Sourcing LinkedIn Thérèse Lever: Psychologist en Libérale.

Director of Studies Professor Malcolm LeGrice: Supervisor of my research on Self-Analysis and the Arts at Central St Martins, University of the Arts London, who encouraged me to write a book and become a lecturer at University.

Dr. Yves Lamontagne for introducing me to Professor Isaac Marks at Maudsley Hospital, part of the Academic Health Science Centre, affiliated with King's College in London, England.

Professor Isaac Marks, who gave me the opportunity to observe and study Behavioural Therapy at Maudsley Hospital, London.

To Jean-Paul Sylvain, a Montréal journalist covering my television work at Télé-Métropole and Radio-Canada, and Terry Tighe, a photographer in London who supported and photographed my research at University. Each of you encouraged and inspired me for my 25-year mission to develop the Zapping therapy as an incredible tool for my followers.

To my husband, Dr. Paul Lelliott, psychiatrist extraordinaire, thank you for all of your support and love.

To Andrée Gagné, social worker, for being my sister.

Contents

Color Your Way to Deeper Transformation

This coloring book illustrates the Zapping Self-Love, Self-Care, and Shiatsu exercises that I've described in more detail in my book, *Zapping: Your Body at Your Service*, and my eBooks, Coloring Books, and e-Coloring Books. By coloring the images, you activate three senses that deepen the transformation you will have from doing the exercises. These three senses are vision, touch, and hearing:

- Vision: Seeing or imagining images of you and others helps create a picture in your mind of what you want to change.

- Touch: Coloring activates a physical response.

- Hearing: Saying affirmations while coloring will integrate the energy into your being.

Each image has a brief description of what to do and say while coloring the parts of the body. The images are of the author doing the described activity; while doing the exercises, imagine that it is your body you are coloring. Filling in the white spaces of the clothing will integrate the information more deeply into your own body.

There may be times when you are not able to physically color the images. When that is the case, you can use a method called "magnetic coloring" to embody in your mind the changes in the exercises that will have a powerful effect. The most significant symbol in each image is the heart. The connection with your heart is the direct link to your brain. By focusing your vision on the hearts in each image, then doing the affirmations and exercises, you can closely simulate the benefits that coloring the images will have.

Zapping refers to a specific position of cupping the hand to access your energetic field for information, combined with clockwise and counterclockwise rotation when using acupressure (based on the Shiatsu self-routine called "Do In"), visualization, and affirmations designed to shift the energy. Your Zapping hand is like a magic wand, your communication access into your inner body. It is the link between your senses and the immediate experience of visualization and affirmation. Your hand in this cupped-hand position transforms you back to your initial state of calmness at a phenomenally fast rate by decluttering unwanted energy and restoring it with self-esteem and self-love.

The exercises in Figures 1.1 – 1.5 are a beautiful routine to do together to begin your day, providing calm and self-love, increasing your happiness and contentment.

Color Zapping in Self-Love

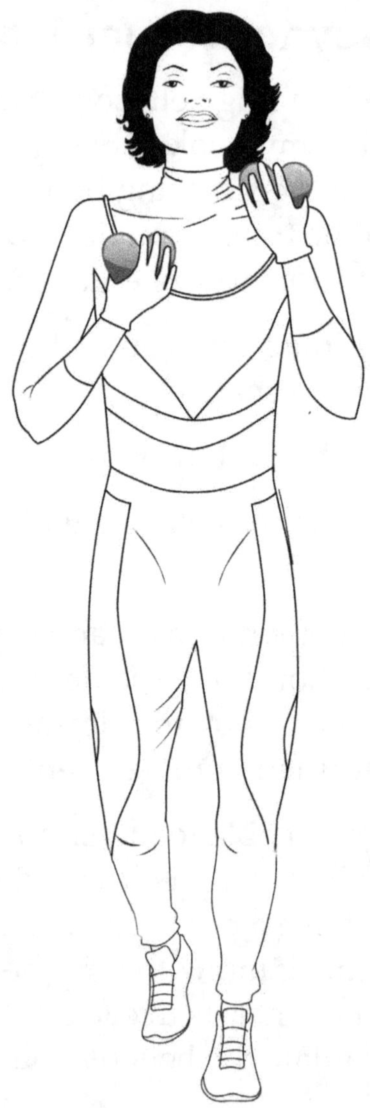

Figure 1.1 – Color Zapping in Self-Love

Zapping in Self-Love is an excellent way to start the day. Take a deep breath and then imagine yourself running forward.

Visualize a red heart in each of your hands. Say to yourself: "I start my day going forward by coloring my body with self-love energy."

Color Zapping in Self-Care

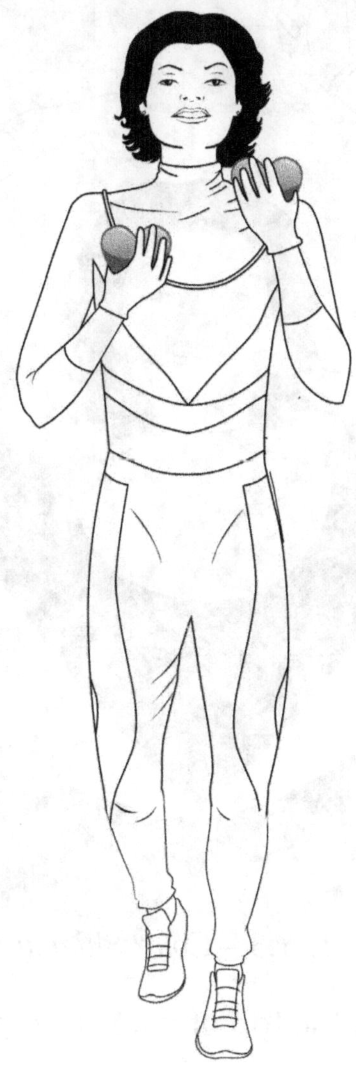

Figure 1.2 – Color Zapping in Self-Care

After coloring yourself running forward, shift to visualizing running backward in the same place, topping off your positive energy.

Visualize one red heart in each hand with the motion of your arms in reverse this time. Say to yourself: "I care for myself in the present and face the day owning my positive, personal energy."

Color Shiatsu Do In

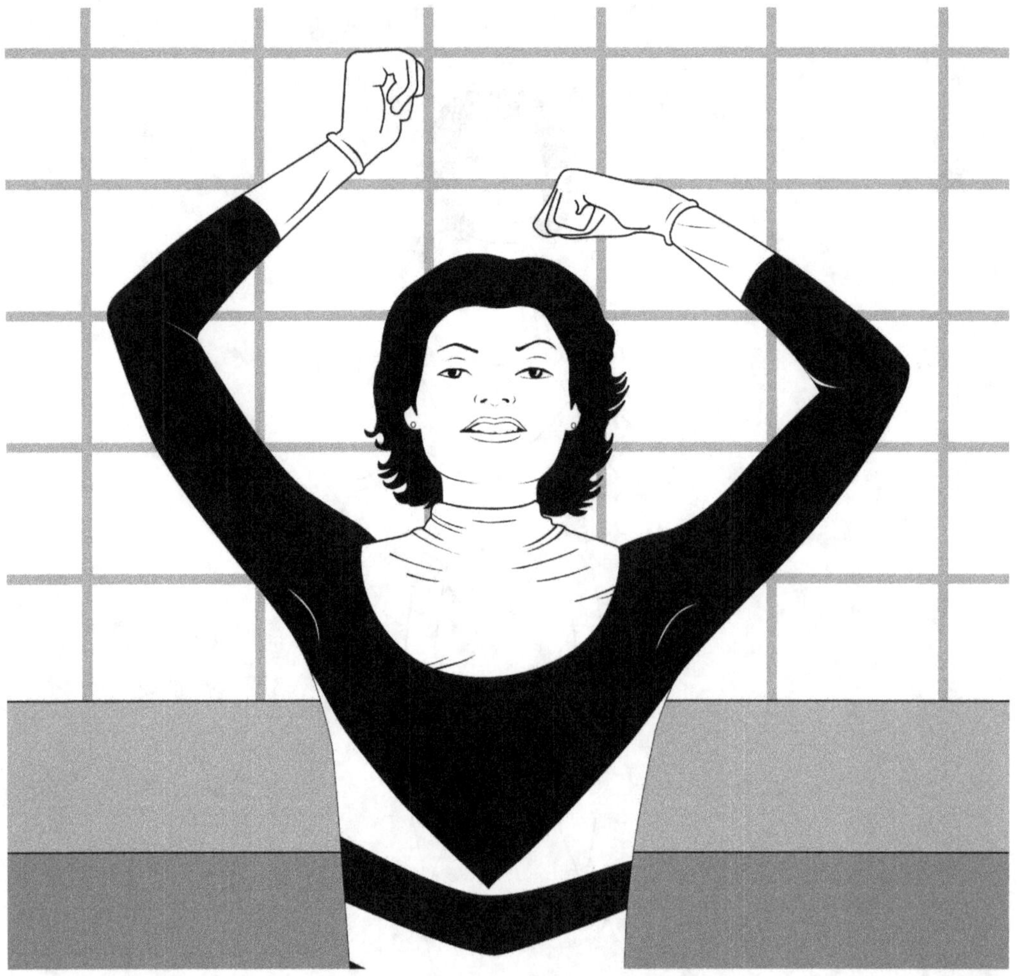

Figure 1.3 – Color Shiatsu Do In

Lightly place your closed fists on the top of your head and gently tap over the crown area.

Take a deep breath and as you are tapping, quietly say, "You are special. You are not alone. I care for you, and I love you." The affirmation reinforces that you are there for yourself, and is particularly effective when you feel upset.

At the end of the exercise, take another deep breath and feel the calm in your body.

Color Daily Habit Routine for Morning and Evening

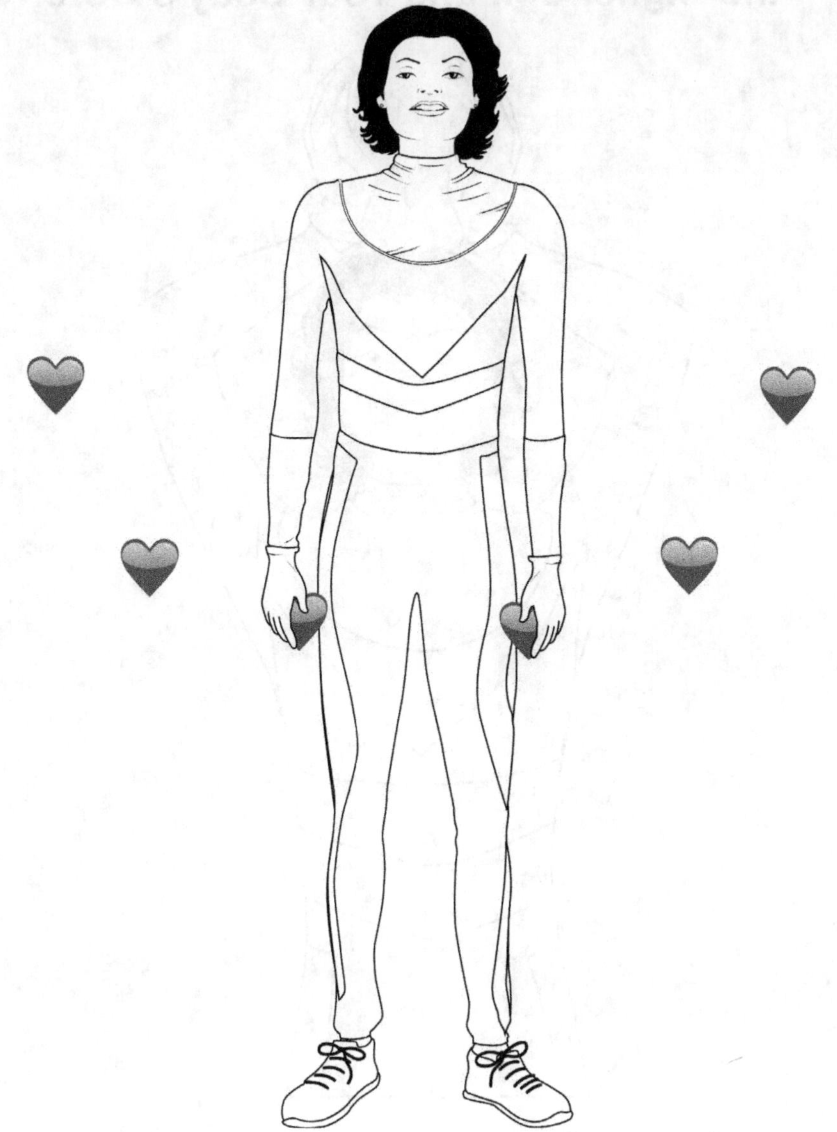

Figure 1.4 – Color Daily Habit Routine for Morning and Evening

Take a deep breath as you visualize and feel a red heart in each hand, and then visualize two more red hearts on each side going upward.

Say quietly to yourself, "I clear my energy, I declutter my energy, and my energy surrounds me. It makes me feel calm. I take my life into my own hands and make sure to live with my own energy. By de-stressing myself calmly and kindly every day, I am my best friend."

Coloring this exercise has an instant calming effect.

Color Being in the Flow of Energy Between the Higher Self and Your Body's Core

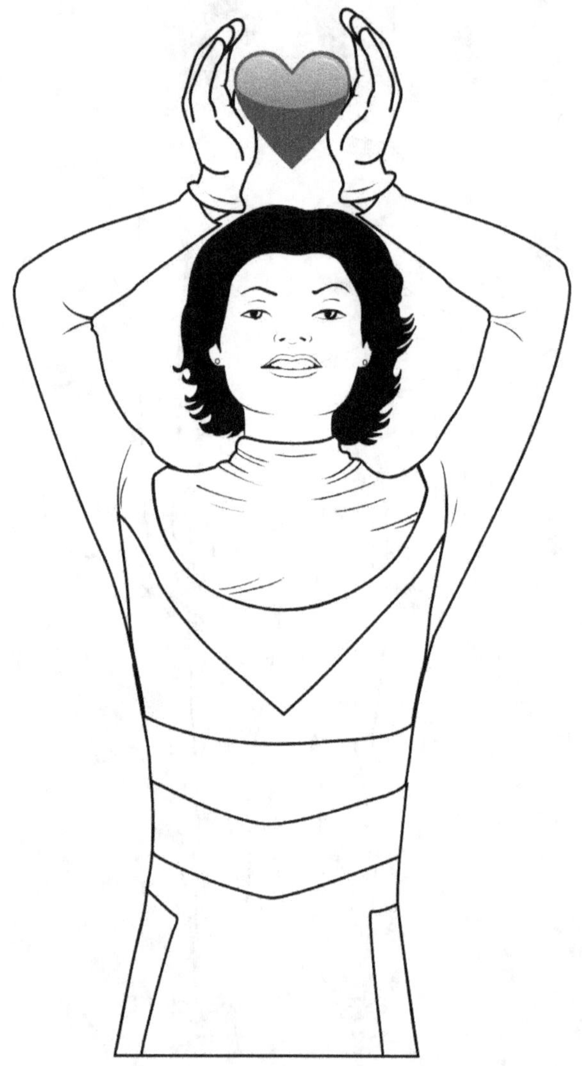

Figure 1.5 – Color Being in the Flow of Energy Between the Higher Self and Your Body's Core

Bring your arms to the top of your head. In the space between your hands, visualize a healthy red heart.

Quietly repeat to yourself the following affirmation: "I am running in the flow of my own energy. I connect easily with my higher energy. I am beautiful."

Daily Home Visualization Exercises to Declutter Your Energy

The following exercises demonstrate how Zapping can declutter a person's energy at home. By sending the transformed energy of love back to anyone whose energy has affected you, you will experience an increase in your energy and relieve stress and fatigue. Often, in the time it takes to take a deep breath of fresh air and get into position for your visualization exercise, you can identify those unconscious sources of your pain.

Color Decluttering Your Body and Sending Energy with Love – Left Side

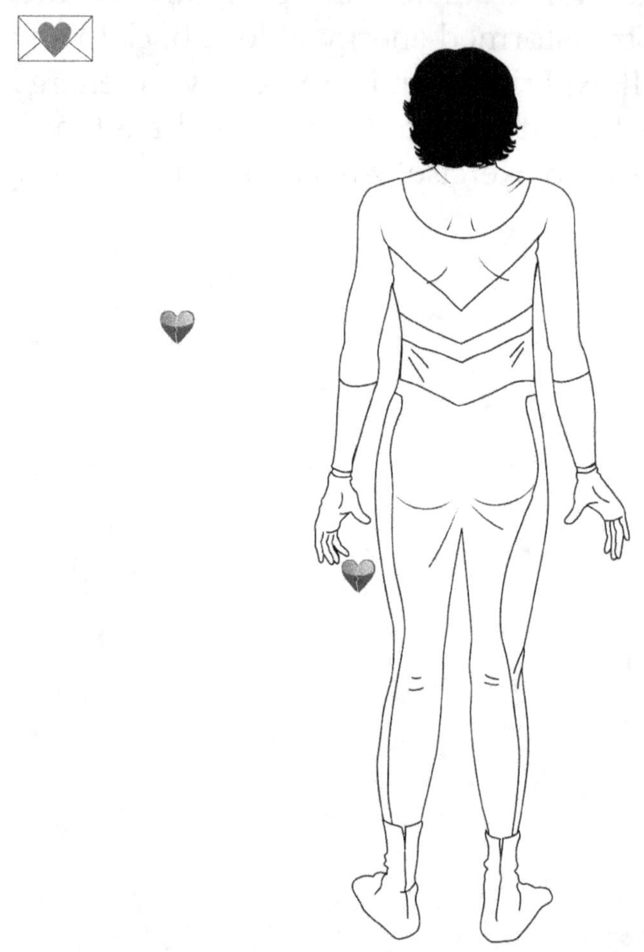

Figure 1.6 – Color Decluttering Your Body and Sending Energy with Love – Left Side

Color sending loving energy back to the person or event that was the source of your discomfort.

Imagine sending a heart envelope, along with an affirmation, to who contributed to your discomfort. For example, the affirmation for your mother might be: "I send my love to you completely, Mother. I love you, and I love myself, and as a result, I am happy to send you this envelope filled with my heart love for you to enjoy."

Color Decluttering Your Body and
Sending Energy with Love – Right Side

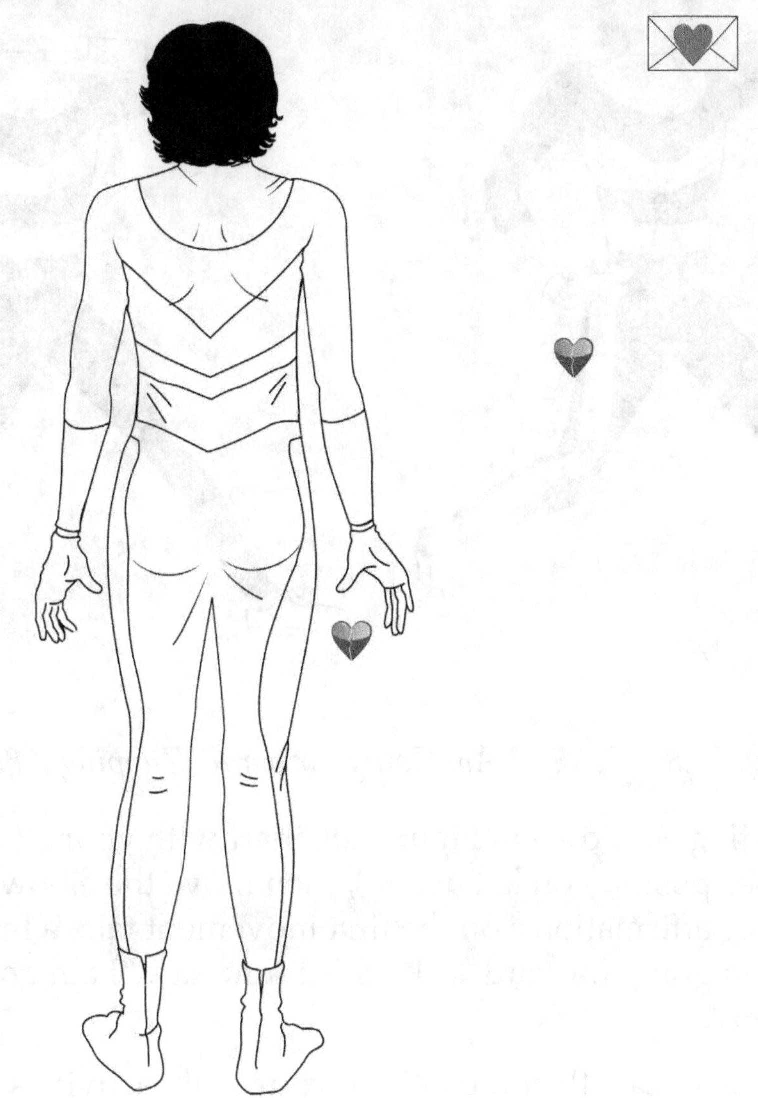

*Figure 1.7 – Color Decluttering Your Body and
Sending Energy with Love – Right Side*

Imagine doing the same decluttering exercise from the right side of your body to rid
yourself of toxins entirely. Each time you send the envelope of love, switch sides to
balance your body.

Color "I Am Going Forward" Zapping Affirmation

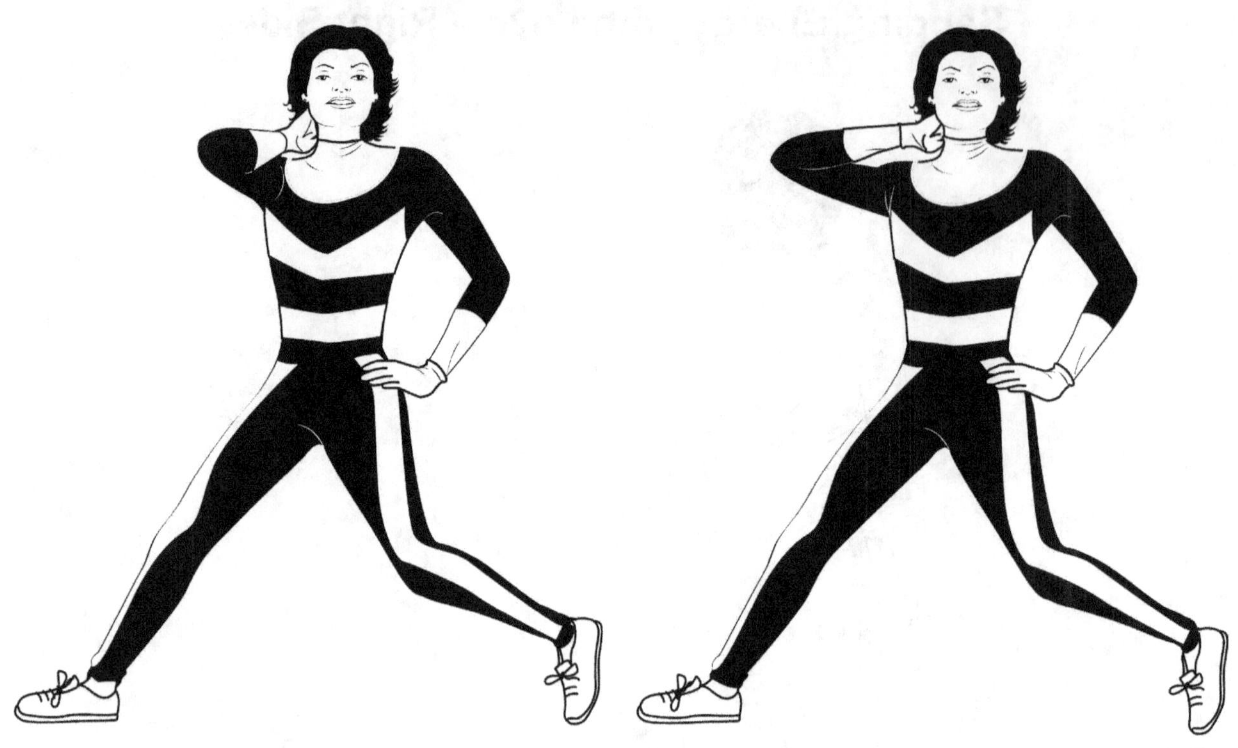

Figure 1.8 – Color "I Am Going Forward" Zapping Affirmation

Color yourself standing as shown in Figure 1.8. Start with your elbow in front of you pointing forward (see position on left above), then move the elbow back and forth as you say the following affirmations: on the first movement take a breath; on the second movement, say, "I am going forward." The third time say, "I am going forward no matter what happens."

Finish with an expansive breath and continue your daily activities.

Color Zapping Aspiring Unconditional Love

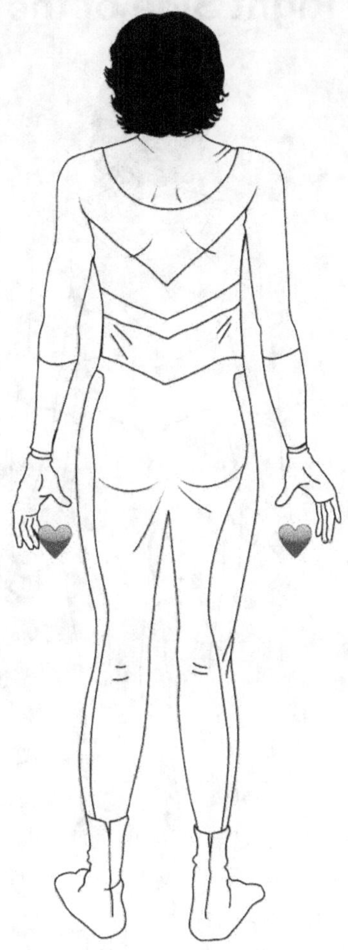

Figure 1.9 – Color Zapping Aspiring Unconditional Love

Color Figure 1.9 while visualizing a red heart inside each hand, suspended between your thumb and index fingers, and imagine energy coming from your higher self into the hearts you are holding.

Say the following affirmations: "I feel love; thank you." Take another breath and say, "I feel that I am love," then take another breath after you say it. When complete, you will feel calm, with a love energy that fills your entire body.

Color Filling with More Unconditional Love:
The Right Side of the Body

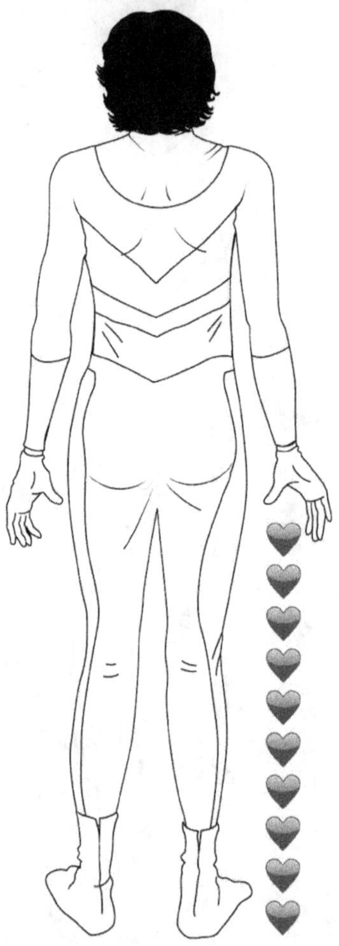

Figure 1.10 – Color Filling with More Unconditional Love:
The Right Side of the Body

While coloring Figure 1.10, take a deep breath. Visualize a row of hearts suspended downward from your right Zapping hand position. Quietly ask your higher self to fill you with unconditional love.

Take a deep breath, then say the following affirmation: "I fill with love from my higher self every day. I receive higher love for my self and others. I feel complete. I am full of love and receive it through my open right hand."

Color Filling with More Unconditional Love:
The Left Side of the Body

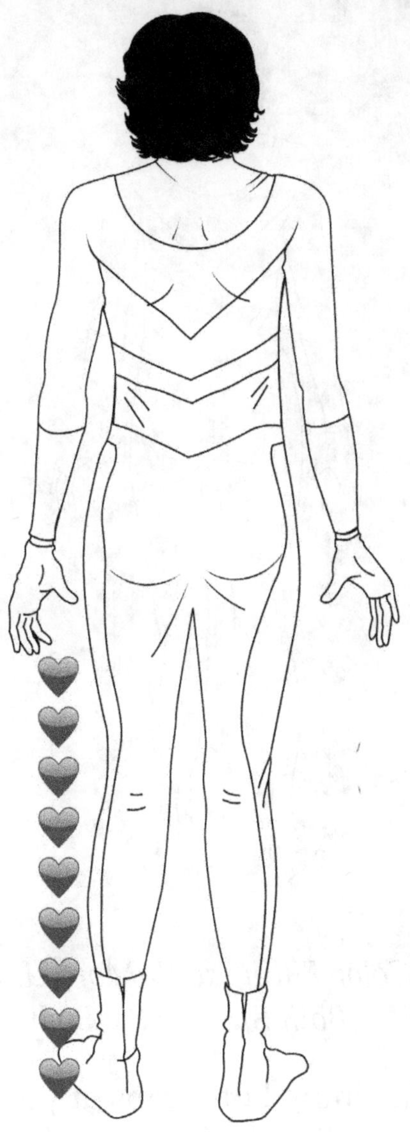

Figure 1.11 – Color Filling with More Unconditional Love:
The Left Side of the Body

While coloring Figure 1.11, take a deep breath as you visualize a row of hearts suspended from your left downward Zapping hand. Breathe deep, and then say the same affirmation as you did for the right side while visualizing the hearts on the left side. You decluttered the left side at the beginning of this series by sending the heart envelopes to their source.

Color Filling with More Unconditional Love:
Both Sides of the Body

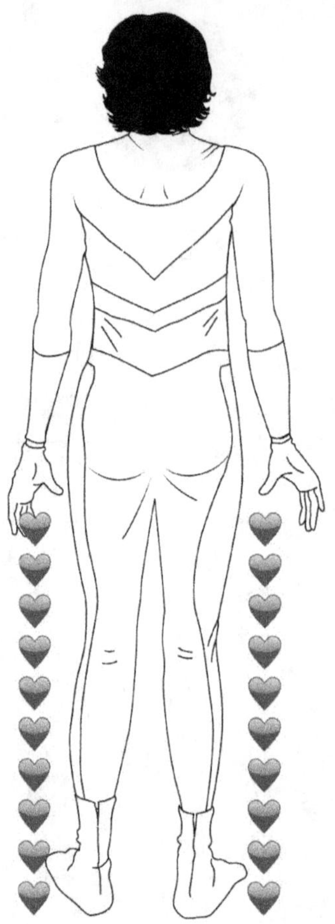

Figure 1.12 – Color Filling with More Unconditional Love:
Both Sides of the Body

Now color Figure 1.12 while imagining both arms at your side and your hands in the downward Zapping position. Visualize the hearts on both sides of your body and the feeling of warmth they give you. Now ask quietly to be filled by self-love.

Ask the higher self: "I ask to receive unconditional love on the right side of my body to fill up the love energy on my left side that I sent to the sources of my pain." See the red hearts take their place, one under the other in a straight line, then transfer to the left side and fill that completely, too. Take a deep breath, and then say, "Fill me with unconditional love so that I feel the wonderful glow of completeness. I feel filled with the warmth of unconditional love that inhabits me."

Color Mindfulness and a Decluttered Body

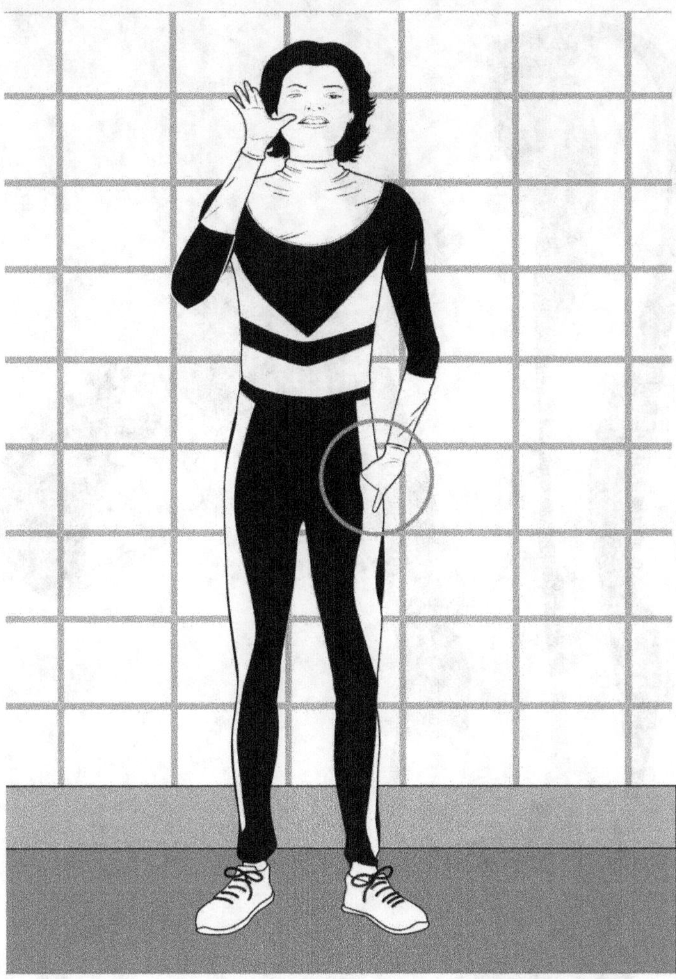

Figure 1.13 – Color Mindfulness and a Decluttered Body

While coloring Figure 1.13, feel yourself in the present moment.

As you continue to color, imagine doing the exercise as described below:

Stand as shown in Figure 1.13. Place your thumb under your right cheekbone with your other fingers open and straight up and your hand facing forward. Close your right eye, keeping your left eye open. With your right thumb, apply a light pressure on the skin and start rotating your thumb in a clockwise direction ten times followed by ten rotations counter-clockwise. Take a deep breath and then do ten rotations in both directions again, followed by another deep breath. Then change sides and do again.

This is a perfect way to break up your day and bring calm to your body.

Color Zapping Stretch with Visualization Affirmation

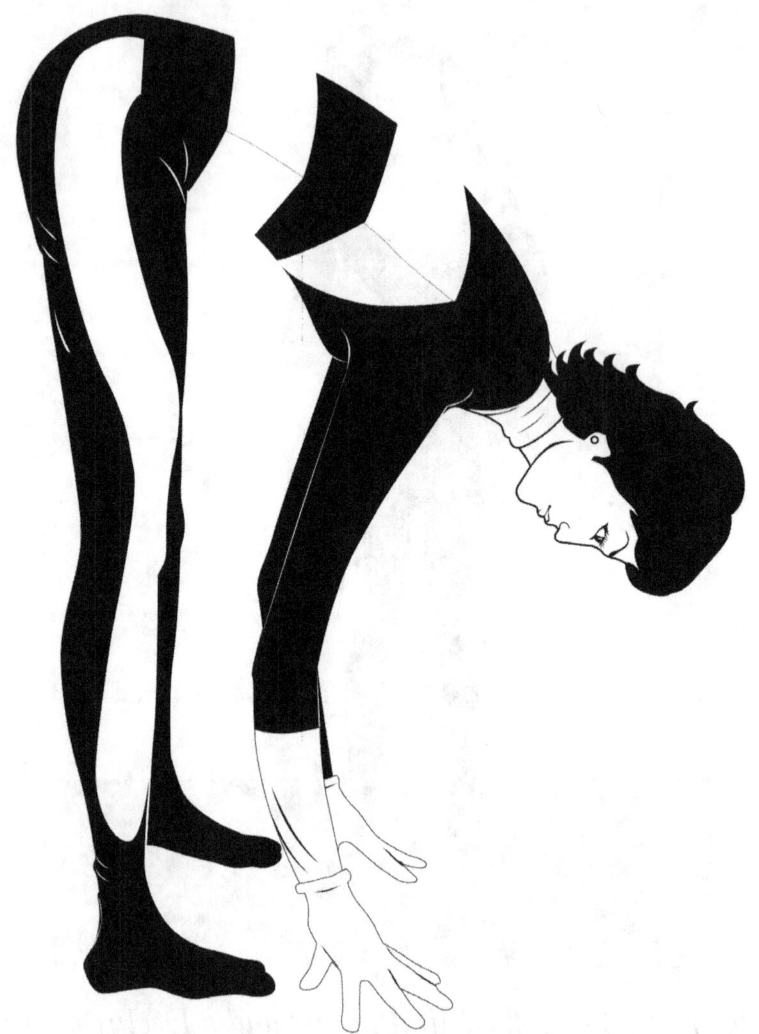

Figure 1.14 – Color Zapping Stretch with Visualization Affirmation

While coloring Figure 1.14, imagine your hands in the Zapping position with your fingers open, and stretching down to the floor. Bring yourself into the present moment and connect with your body.

Take a deep breath and say quietly to yourself: "I am the caregiver of my body. I start the day by telling myself in the present moment, 'Dear body, I will supervise my activities for today, taking breaks when necessary to not over stress you. I will cherish and fill you with Zapping self-love, doing a full stretch routine to give you breaks during the day. I am dedicated to you.'"

Color "Yes, I Love My Body" Stretch

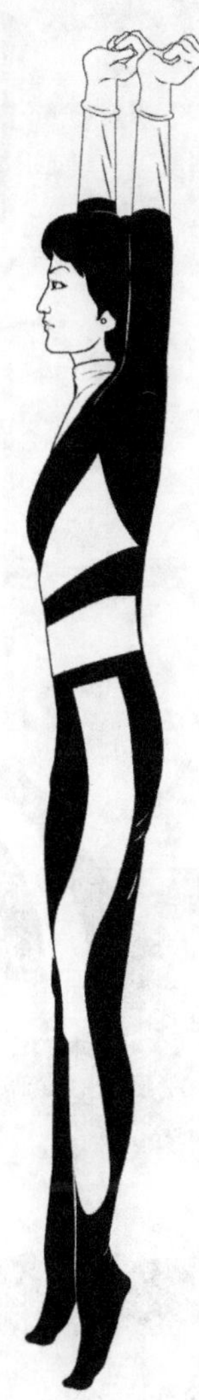

Figure 1.15 – Color "Yes, I Love My Body" Stretch

Imagine as you color that you are stretching upward with your arms straight above your head and standing on your toes. Take a deep breath, and then imagine closing your fists.

Now visualize your fists opening as you say the following affirmation: "I am the caregiver of my body. It is the start of the day, and I'm telling you dear body that I will take care of you by giving you the breaks necessary to not be overwhelmed by stress. I will cherish special moments during the day with my Zapping stretch routine."

Color Opening Your Heart to Liberation

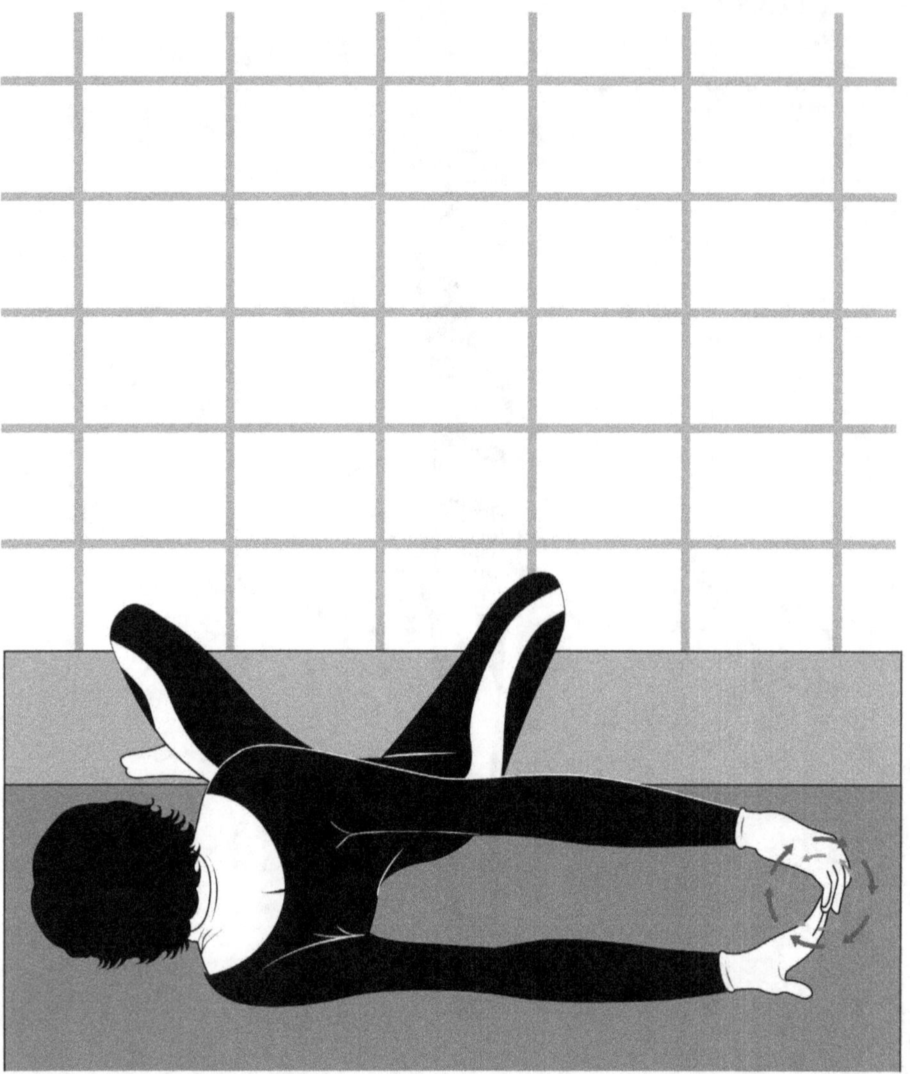

Figure 1.16 – Color Opening Your Heart to Liberation

As you color, imagine being in the position demonstrated in Figure 1.16, with the fingers of each hand touching while in the Zapping position. Visualize doing the exercise: make a very light circular movement (see the arrows in Figure 1.16). Do a set of ten clockwise followed by a set of 10 counter-clockwise, allowing your body to relax and your energy to flow openly.

As you continue to visualize remaining on the floor on your side as your body relaxes into the position, take a nice, serene, fresh breath before silently saying to yourself the following affirmation: "I feel good. I am in the present moment. I am love."

Color Decluttering Your Life and Restoring Self-Love

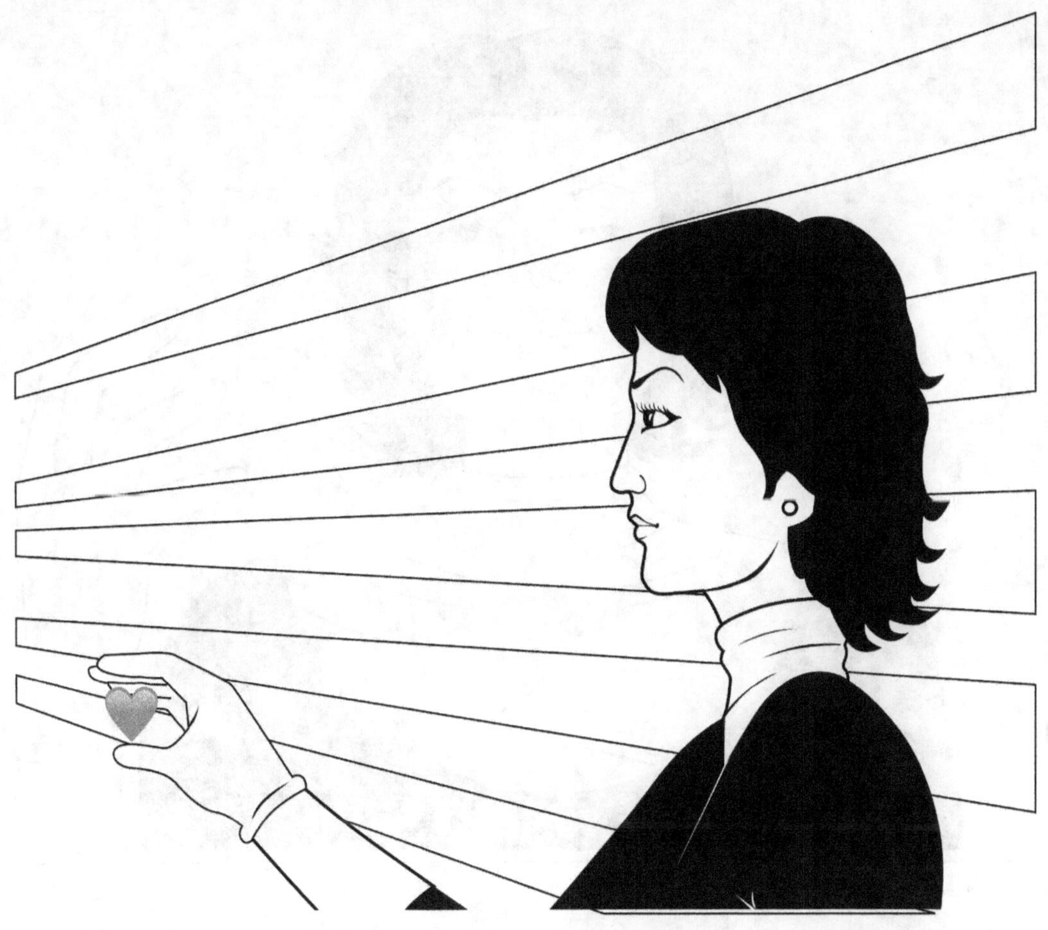

Figure 1.17 – Color Decluttering Your Life and Restoring Self-Love

As you color Figure 1.17, imagine standing in front of a window looking outside. Direct your Zapping hand to the window as you look straight ahead.

Take a deep, expansive breath and visualize the heart in the inside of your hand as you say to yourself the following affirmation: "I love my brain [your name]. I have the capability and willingness to go inside my body and breathe consciously. Let self-love inhabit me. I feel full of self-love in my body. I declutter the pain that I feel at the moment."

Color Creating a New Mindset Using Zapping

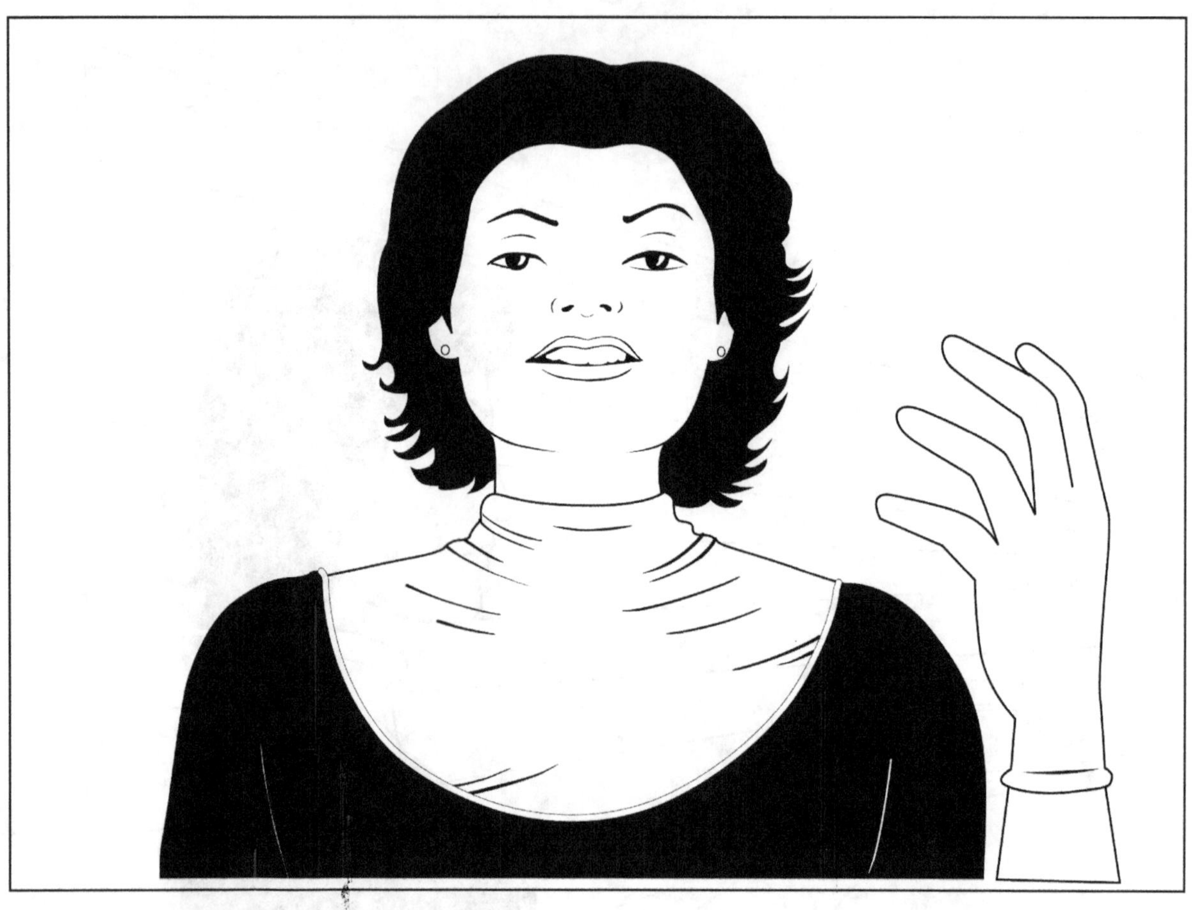

Figure 1.18 – Color Creating a New Mindset Using Zapping

Color Figure 1.18 while visualizing yourself bringing your hand up and curving your fingers slightly inward, leaving space in your palm as if you were holding a soft ball. In this position, the hand has a fantastic ability to communicate with your body and bring self-love, self-esteem, gratitude, and calmness to both body and mind.

Take a deep breath and say the following affirmation: "The soft, warm feeling in the middle of my hand is how I fill my body with warmth every day."

Color Engaging Your Body During Affirmations

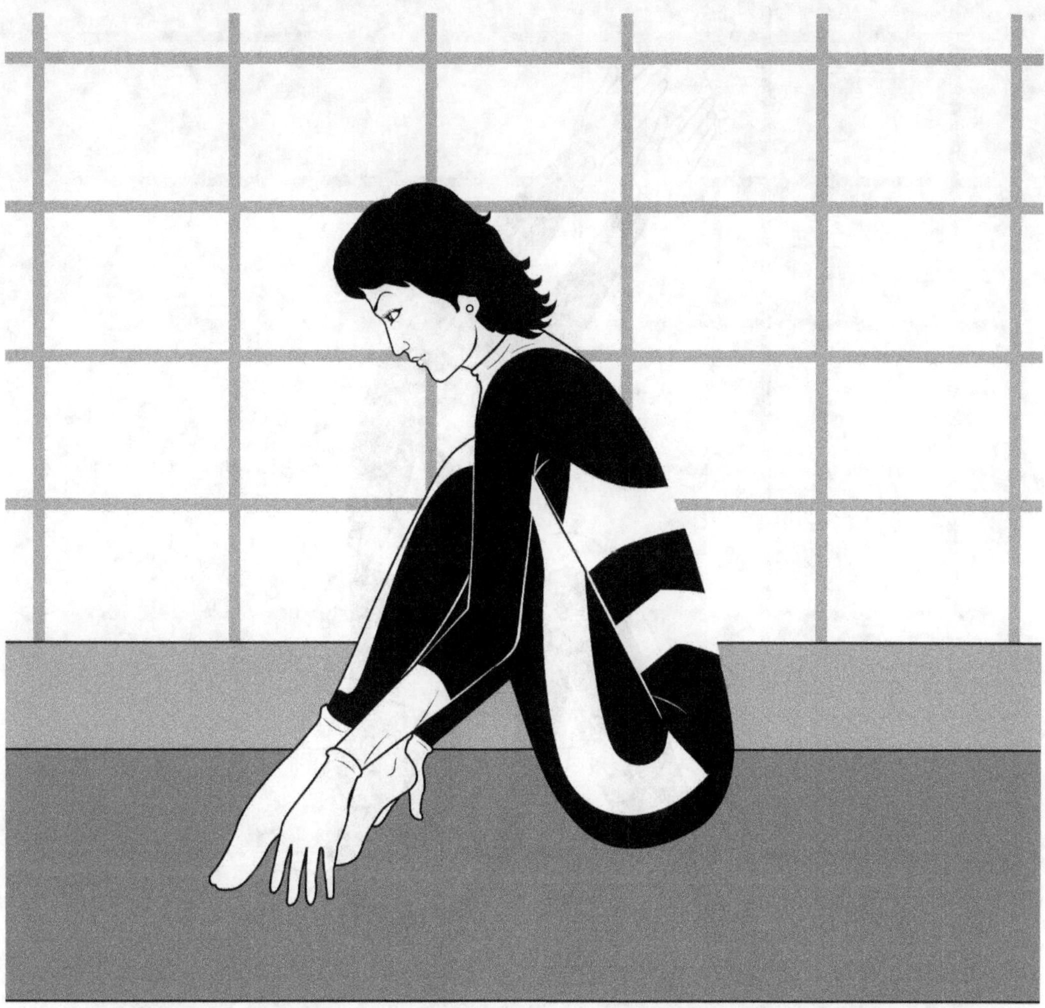

Figure 1.19 – Color Engaging Your Body During Affirmations

Figures 1.19 – 1.21 are a series of coloring pictures to help you quickly alleviate any feelings of emptiness in your inner self.

Color Figure 1.19 while imagining being in the position shown. With your eyes focused down and your fingers and toes touching the floor, imagine a deep contact with the earth, while being conscious of your body. Salute the energy that your body takes from the earth when eating or exercising or walking on it.

Say the following affirmation: "The good and healthy food I eat and exercises I do on earth fill my inner body with warm energy that fills me up."

Color Going Within Your Body

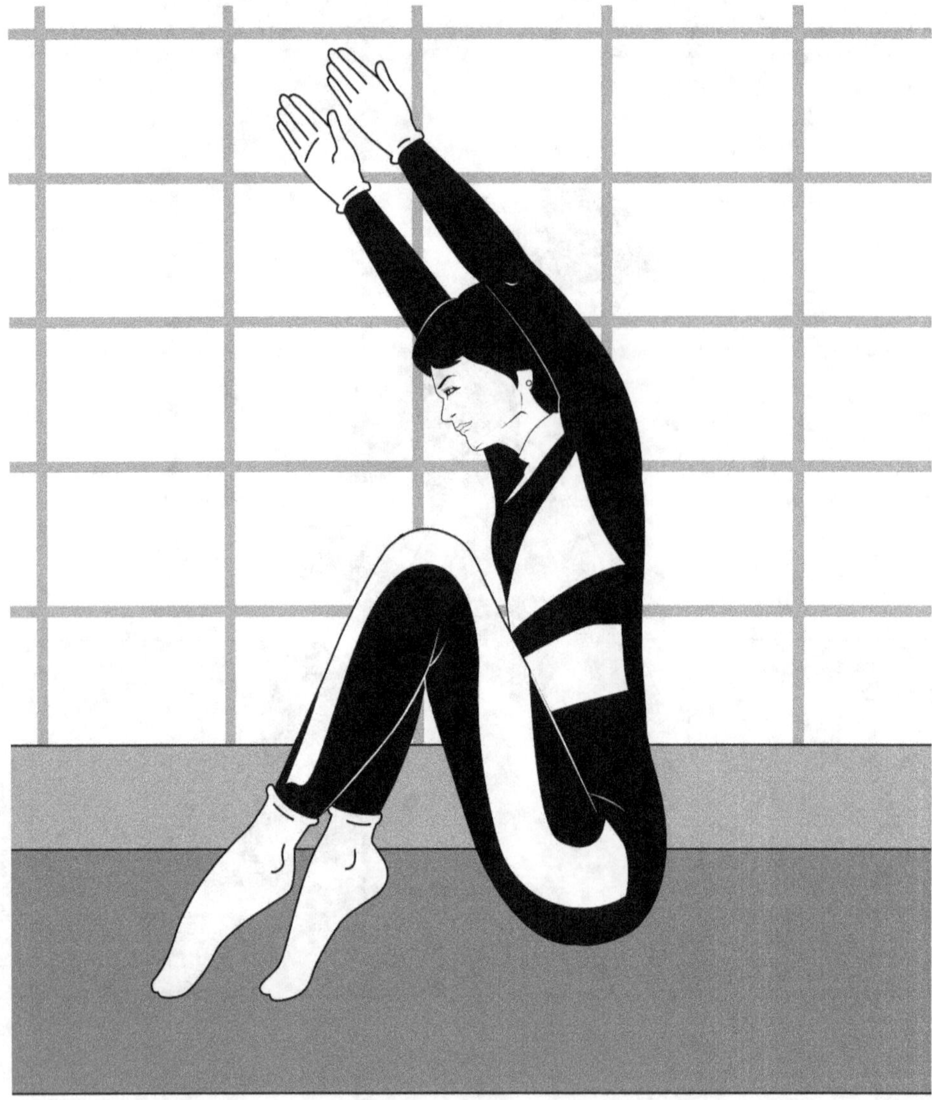

Figure 1.20 – Color Going Within Your Body

Now color Figure 1.20 as you imagine staying in the same position while elevating your arms and stretching to the maximum position possible. Salute your inner connection to earth. Inhale, and then exhale while connecting the energy from your heart to your higher self.

Say the affirmation: "My inner self is full of loving energy. I feel complete and connected to my space and energy."

This exercise helps to keep your body healthy and your mind positive.

Color the Fusion of Head and Body
in Affirmation Body Exercises

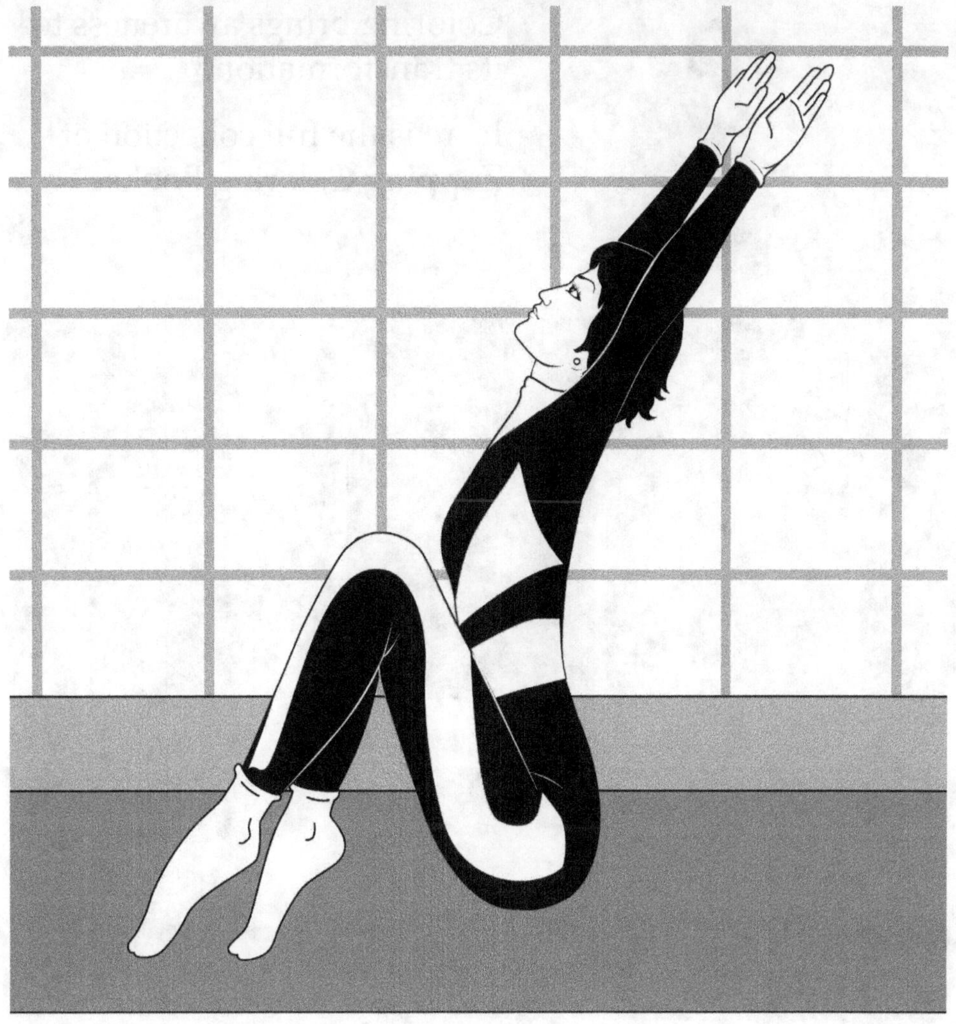

Figure 1.21 – Color the Fusion of Head and Body in Affirmation Body Exercises

Continue to imagine being in the same position, feeling the fusion of head and body with the energy below and above you, and shifting your arms and stretching backward as shown above.

As you color Figure 1.21, connect with the energy within you, then open and close your eyes while saying the following affirmation: "I am grounded, calm, and centered in all parts of my body." Color the image to reinforce the power of your inner calm.

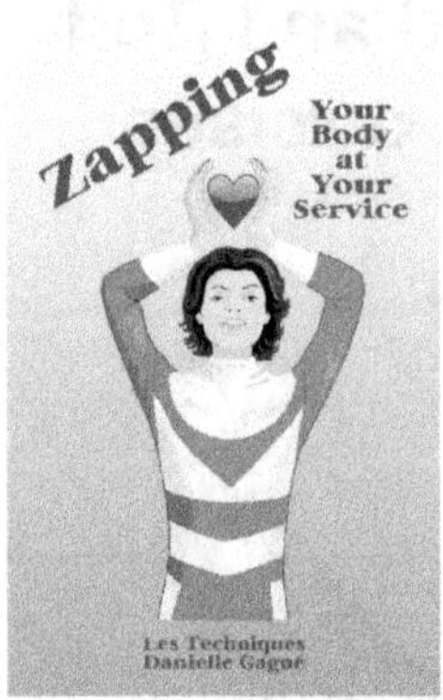

Your Body is Precious!

Coloring brings awareness to its transformation.

Here is the full collection of Zapping Coloring Books…

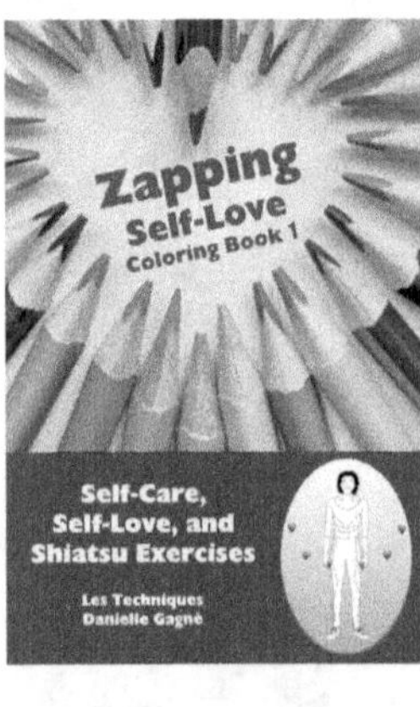

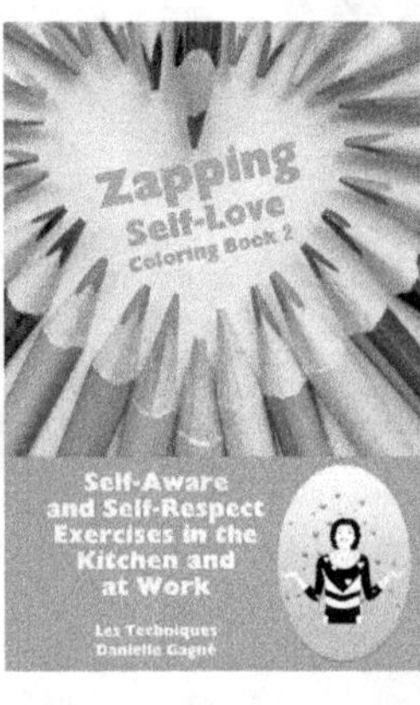

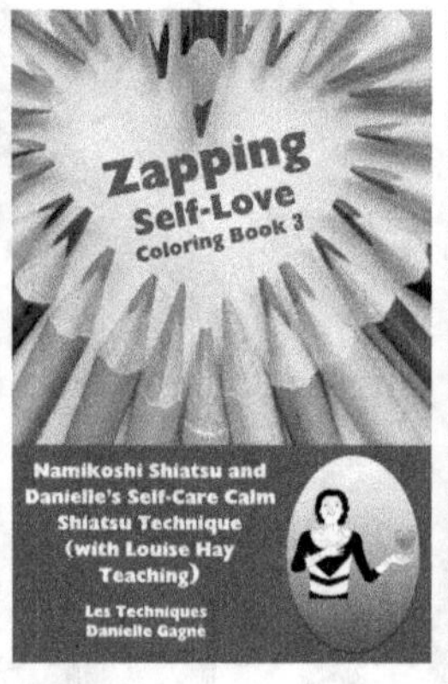

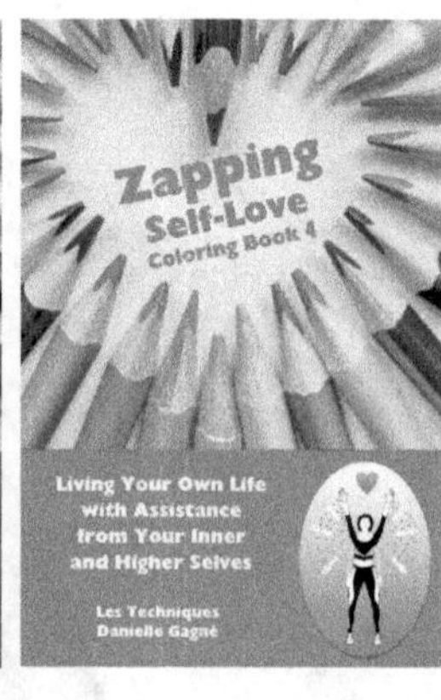

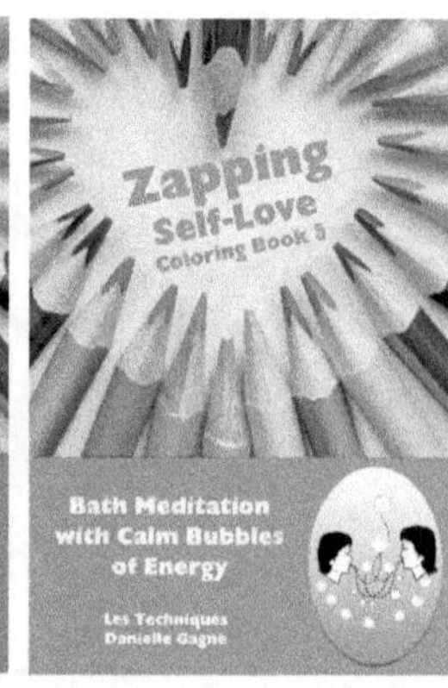

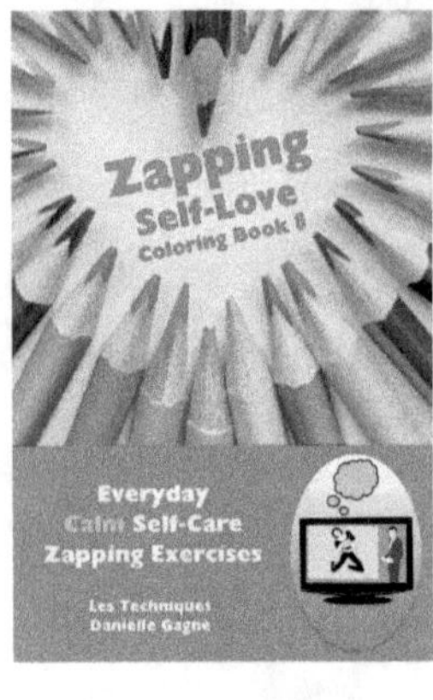

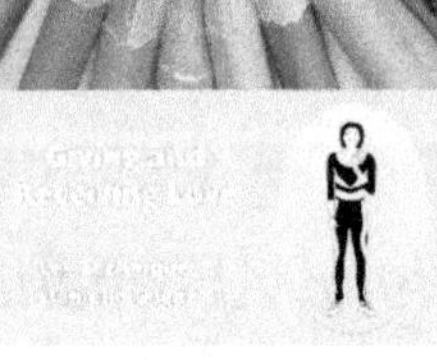

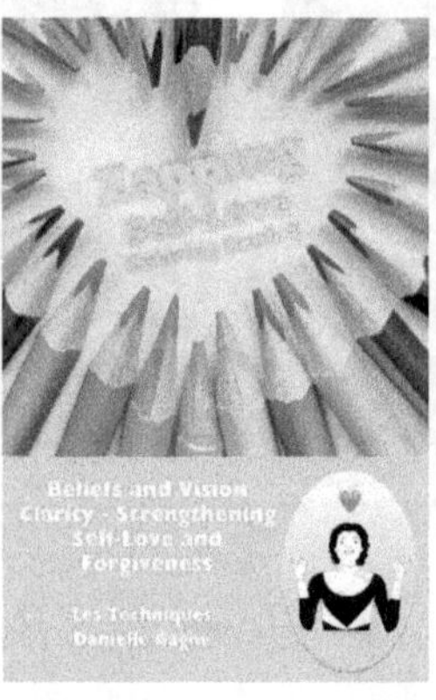

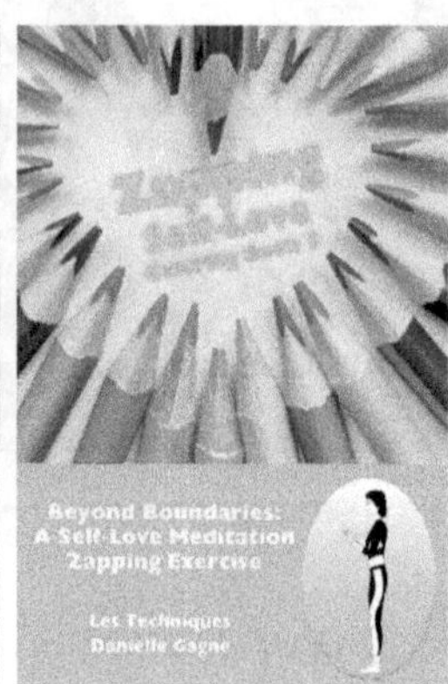

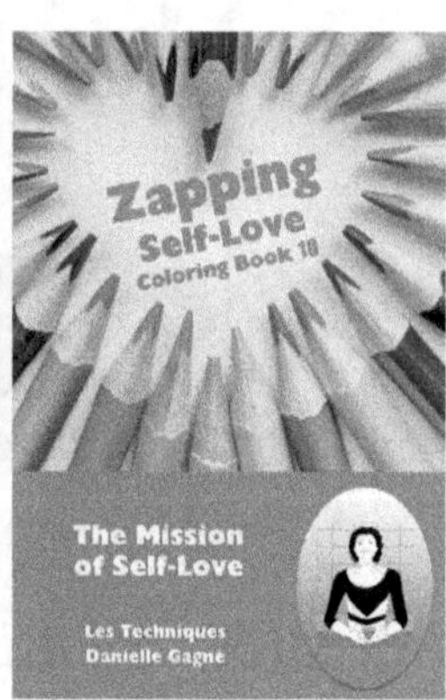

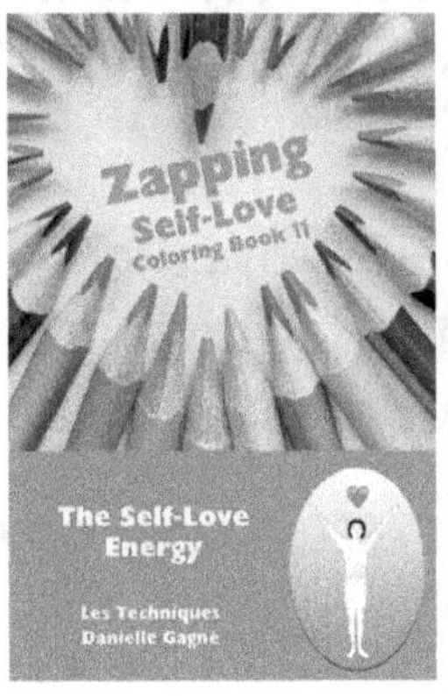

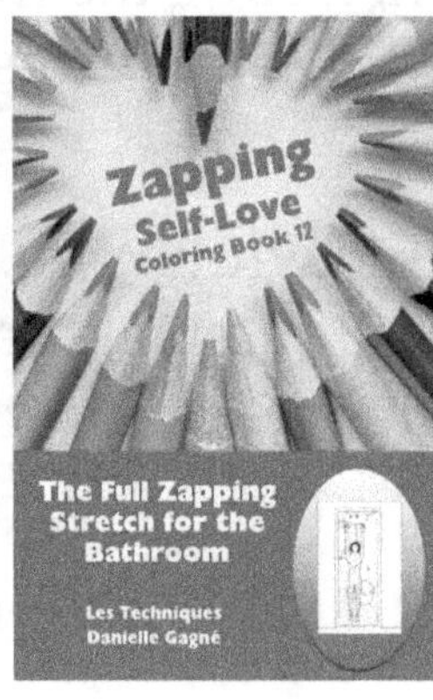

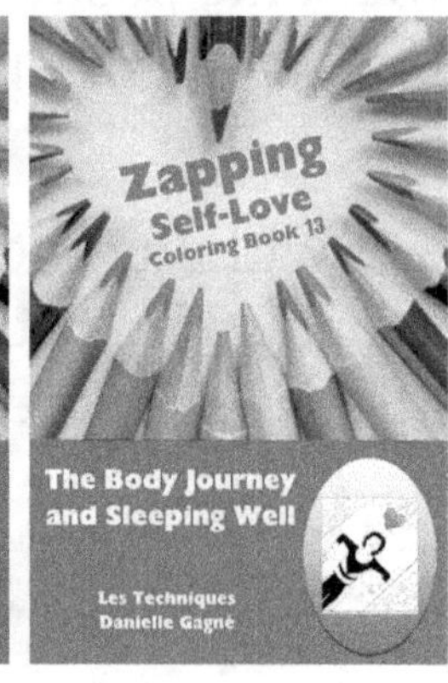

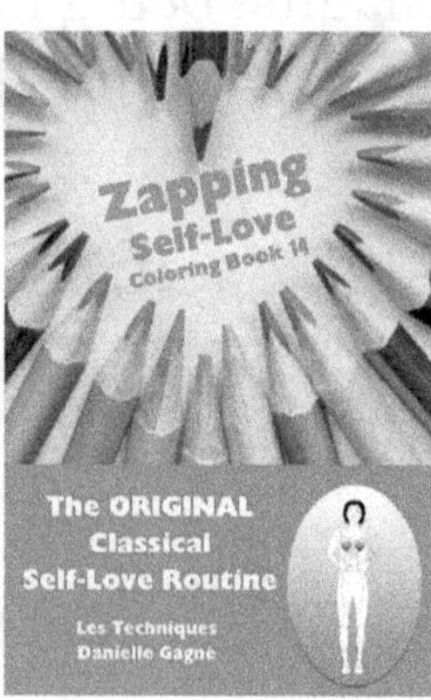

www.ingramcontent.com/pod-product-compliance
Lightning Source LLC
Chambersburg PA
CBHW081257250726
48654CB00012B/1638